Bone Fitness Handbook

Secret to Stronger, Healthier Bones

BY

Dr. Linda Jefferson

Copyright

No part of this book should be copied, reproduced without the author's permission © 2023

TABLE OF CONTENT

INTRODUCTION

Osteoporosis, a silent yet formidable adversary, is a medical condition characterized by the gradual weakening of bones, rendering them porous and more susceptible to fractures. Derived from the Greek words "osteo" (bone) and "porosis" (porous), the term encapsulates the essence of the disease—progressive bone loss leading to diminished density and strength. Bones, dynamic and living tissues, undergo a perpetual cycle of breakdown and renewal. However, in osteoporosis, this equilibrium is disrupted as bone resorption surpasses the rate of new bone formation.

The consequences of osteoporosis extend beyond the skeletal system, impacting overall health and quality of life. More prevalent in aging populations, especially postmenopausal women due to hormonal shifts, it also affects men and younger individuals with specific risk factors. Though often asymptomatic in its early stages, the insidious nature of osteoporosis manifests in heightened fracture susceptibility, particularly in weight-bearing bones like the spine, hip, and wrist.

Understanding osteoporosis involves delving into its intricacies—the interplay of genetics, lifestyle choices, and hormonal influences. A comprehensive grasp of this condition is essential for both prevention and effective management, emphasizing the significance of bone health as a foundation for a vibrant and resilient life.

The Basics of Bone Health

The basics of bone health lie at the core of our physical well-being, as bones serve as the structural framework for the body, providing support, protection, and facilitating movement. Bone health is a dynamic process influenced by a delicate equilibrium between bone formation and resorption. Bones are composed of a dense network of minerals, primarily calcium and phosphorus, embedded in a collagen matrix, rendering them both strong and flexible.

Crucial to bone health is the continuous cycle of remodeling, where old or damaged bone is broken down and replaced by new, healthy bone tissue. This intricate dance is orchestrated by osteoblasts, responsible for bone formation, and osteoclasts, tasked with bone resorption. The mineralization process, facilitated by minerals such as calcium, fortifies bone structure and density.

The foundation for optimal bone health is laid in early life, with childhood and adolescence representing critical periods for bone development. Adequate nutrition, particularly calcium and vitamin D intake, along with weight-bearing exercises, play pivotal roles in fostering robust bone growth. As individuals age, maintaining bone health becomes increasingly vital, necessitating a holistic approach that incorporates nutrition, physical activity, and lifestyle choices to fortify this essential scaffolding that supports a healthy and active life.

Impact of Osteoporosis on Daily Life

The impact of osteoporosis on daily life is profound, often transforming routine activities into potential hazards. This insidious condition, characterized by weakened bones, manifests its consequences in heightened fracture risk, especially in weight-bearing areas like the spine, hips, and wrists. Individuals grappling with osteoporosis encounter a pervasive fear of fractures, influencing their daily choices and movements.

Simple tasks, such as bending, lifting, or even a minor fall, become sources of apprehension as the risk of fractures looms large. The spine, a common site of osteoporotic fractures, may undergo compression fractures, leading to pain, diminished height, and a stooped posture, impacting one's self-image and physical functionality. Hip fractures, another prevalent outcome, often result in reduced mobility, increased dependence, and a higher likelihood of complications.

Beyond the physical toll, the emotional and psychological impact of osteoporosis is substantial. Chronic pain, fear of fractures, and limitations in mobility contribute to a sense of vulnerability and can lead to social withdrawal. Daily life becomes a delicate balance between preserving independence and mitigating the risk of injury.

The ripple effect extends to familial and social spheres, necessitating adjustments and support systems. The holistic impact of osteoporosis on daily life underscores the urgency of proactive measures in bone health, emphasizing prevention, early detection, and comprehensive management to mitigate its pervasive effects.

Scope and Importance of the Book

This book on osteoporosis holds a paramount significance in bridging the knowledge gap and fostering a comprehensive understanding of a condition that silently jeopardizes bone health. Its scope extends far beyond mere medical insights, reaching out to a diverse audience that includes individuals unfamiliar with osteoporosis, those seeking preventive measures, and those currently grappling with the challenges of its management.

For those unacquainted with osteoporosis, this book serves as an informative guide, unraveling the intricacies of bone health, the development of osteoporosis, and its potential ramifications. It transforms complex medical concepts into accessible knowledge, empowering readers to make informed decisions about their health.

Concurrently, the book addresses the needs of individuals keen on preventive strategies. By delving into lifestyle modifications, dietary choices, and early detection methods, it offers a roadmap to fortify bone health proactively. The emphasis on holistic well-being underscores the book's commitment to empowering readers to take charge of their bone health throughout their lifespan.

Equally vital is the book's role as a detailed companion for those already contending with osteoporosis. By providing nuanced insights into medical treatments, dietary factors, and strategies for maintaining quality of life, it becomes a valuable resource for individuals navigating the challenges of this condition.

In essence, the book encapsulates the holistic scope and importance of promoting bone health, ensuring that its readers not only comprehend osteoporosis but are also equipped with the tools to prevent, manage, and thrive despite its challenges.

Who Should Read This Book?

This book is crafted for a diverse audience, catering to individuals at various stages of familiarity and engagement with osteoporosis. It beckons those unfamiliar with the condition, offering a clear and accessible entry point into the world of bone health. Readers seeking preventive measures will find valuable insights, as the book provides a roadmap for fortifying bone health through lifestyle choices, nutrition, and early detection strategies.

For those currently grappling with osteoporosis, the book becomes an indispensable companion, offering detailed explanations of medical treatments, dietary considerations, and strategies for maintaining a fulfilling life while managing the challenges posed by weakened bones. Caregivers, family members, and friends supporting individuals with osteoporosis will also find this book invaluable, gaining a deeper understanding of the condition and how to provide effective assistance and encouragement.

Healthcare professionals, including doctors, nurses, and nutritionists, will discover a comprehensive resource to augment their knowledge and aid in patient education. Researchers and academics delving into bone health will appreciate the synthesis of current knowledge and emerging trends in osteoporosis research.

In essence, this book is a versatile guide, extending its reach to anyone interested in preserving or enhancing their bone health, from the curious novice to the seasoned healthcare professional, fostering a shared commitment to proactive bone care and overall well-being.

CHAPTER ONE

Anatomy of Bones

The anatomy of bones is a marvel of intricacy, representing the structural foundation of the human body. Bones, dynamic and living tissues, provide essential support, protection, and a framework for bodily movement. Comprising a complex matrix of minerals, primarily calcium and phosphorus, woven into a collagen network, bones achieve a delicate balance between strength and flexibility.

Understanding bone anatomy involves exploring its hierarchical structure. At the macroscopic level, long bones, such as the femur and humerus, feature a shaft (diaphysis) and extremities (epiphyses), with a medullary cavity housing marrow. Compact bone forms the dense outer layer, while spongy bone, with its trabeculae, resides within.

Moving inward, microscopic examination reveals the basic functional units—osteons. These cylindrical structures contain concentric layers of mineralized matrix and osteocytes, interconnected by canaliculi facilitating nutrient exchange. Osteoblasts, responsible for bone formation, and osteoclasts, orchestrating resorption, operate within this dynamic microenvironment.

The significance of bone anatomy extends beyond its mechanical role. Bones are sites of hematopoiesis, producing blood cells in the marrow. Additionally, they act as reservoirs for essential minerals, contributing to systemic homeostasis. In essence, the anatomy of bones is a testament to the body's ingenuity, harmonizing strength, resilience, and adaptability in this fundamental framework.

Understanding Bone Structure

Understanding bone structure is paramount in unraveling the intricate framework that supports our bodies. Bones, far from being inert, are dynamic structures undergoing constant remodeling and adaptation. Composed of both organic and inorganic components, the unique architecture of bones provides strength, flexibility, and a reservoir for essential minerals.

At the macroscopic level, bones exhibit two main types: compact and spongy. Compact bone forms the dense outer layer, offering strength and protection, while spongy bone, arranged in a lattice-like structure, provides resilience and reduces overall weight. This dual composition is particularly evident in long bones, where the diaphysis and epiphyses showcase distinct characteristics.

Microscopically, the structural unit of compact bone is the osteon or Haversian system. Osteons consist of concentric lamellae surrounding a central canal, housing blood vessels and nerves. Interconnected by canaliculi, these structures facilitate the exchange of nutrients and waste products between osteocytes, the bone cells residing in lacunae.

Understanding bone structure involves acknowledging the vital roles of osteoblasts, responsible for bone formation, and osteoclasts, orchestrating bone resorption. This dynamic equilibrium ensures the continuous renewal of bone tissue. Appreciating the intricacies of bone structure not only unveils the elegance of the skeletal system but also underscores the adaptability and resilience inherent in maintaining the integrity of this essential anatomical foundation.

The Bone Remodeling Process

The bone remodeling process is a sophisticated dance of cellular activities that ensures the constant renewal and adaptation of bone tissue throughout the human lifespan. This dynamic mechanism is orchestrated by two key players: osteoblasts and osteoclasts, working in harmony to maintain the delicate balance between bone formation and resorption.

Osteoblasts are the architects of the process, responsible for synthesizing and depositing new bone matrix. They meticulously lay down collagen fibers and mineralize them with calcium and phosphorus, contributing to the structural integrity of bones. In contrast, osteoclasts are the demolition crew, specialized cells that break down and absorb old or damaged bone tissue through a process known as resorption.

The bone remodeling process occurs continuously in small packets called basic multicellular units (BMUs). Each BMU involves the coordinated activity of osteoblasts and osteoclasts, ensuring that bone formation keeps pace with resorption. This orchestrated ballet of cellular activities serves several crucial purposes, including repairing micro-damage, adapting bone structure to mechanical stresses, and maintaining the optimal mineral composition of bones.

Factors such as hormonal signals, mechanical loading, and the body's need for calcium regulation influence the bone remodeling process. This dynamic cycle underscores the remarkable adaptability and resilience of the skeletal system, essential for maintaining bone health and responding to the ever-changing demands placed upon it. Understanding the intricacies of bone remodeling provides insights into the resilience and continual adaptation that characterize this vital aspect of human physiology.

The Dynamic Nature of Bones

The dynamic nature of bones is a testament to their perpetual adaptation and responsiveness to the ever-changing demands placed on the human body. Unlike static structures, bones are living tissues engaged in a continuous cycle of remodeling, a process vital for maintaining strength, integrity, and functionality.

At the heart of this dynamism are two key cell types: osteoblasts and osteoclasts. Osteoblasts, the architects of bone formation, synthesize organic matrix and facilitate its mineralization, contributing to bone density and structure. In contrast, osteoclasts are specialized cells responsible for resorption, breaking down and absorbing old or damaged bone tissue.

The intricate balance between osteoblast and osteoclast activity ensures that bones remain adaptive throughout life. Mechanical loading, hormonal signals, and the body's need for calcium regulation influence this dynamic equilibrium. Bones respond to external forces by adjusting their structure, a phenomenon essential for maintaining optimal strength and functionality.

The dynamic nature of bones is particularly evident in their ability to repair micro-damage and adapt to changing mechanical stresses. This adaptability is crucial for accommodating growth during development, responding to changes in physical activity, and healing after injuries. Understanding and appreciating the dynamic nature of bones underscores their role not only as a static structural framework but as a resilient and responsive part of the intricate machinery of the human body.

Bone Growth and Development

Bone growth and development represent a marvel of biological orchestration, shaping the skeletal framework from infancy through adulthood. The process, known as ossification, involves the transformation of cartilage or connective tissue into bone, giving rise to the intricate and dynamic structure that supports the human body.

During early development, bones form through two main methods: intramembranous ossification and endochondral ossification. Intramembranous ossification occurs when bone forms directly within connective tissue membranes, contributing to the development of flat bones like the skull. Endochondral ossification, on the other hand, involves the replacement of cartilage with bone tissue and is responsible for the formation of long bones, such as those in the limbs.

Throughout childhood and adolescence, bones undergo a phase of rapid growth, driven by the activity of growth plates located near the ends of long bones. These growth plates are sensitive to hormonal signals, particularly growth hormone and sex hormones, which regulate the rate and duration of bone growth. Adequate nutrition, including calcium, phosphorus, and vitamin D, plays a pivotal role in supporting this developmental process.

The culmination of bone growth typically occurs by the end of adolescence, as growth plates close, marking the completion of longitudinal growth. Understanding the intricacies of bone growth and development unveils the biological symphony that shapes the foundation of the human body and underscores the importance of nurturing bone health from an early age.

The Lifelong Journey of Bone Health

The journey of bone health is a lifelong odyssey, marked by distinct phases that shape the skeletal system from infancy through the golden years. Commencing at birth, the skeletal foundation undergoes rapid development and growth, driven by genetic factors and environmental influences. Nutrition, particularly the intake of calcium, phosphorus, and vitamin D, plays a pivotal role during these formative years, laying the groundwork for optimal bone density.

Childhood and adolescence constitute a critical chapter in the saga of bone health, marked by the active growth of bones and the presence of growth plates. Hormonal influences, including growth hormone and sex hormones, guide the pace and duration of bone growth. It is during this period that lifestyle choices, such as regular physical activity, contribute to building strong bones and establishing habits that endure into adulthood.

As adulthood unfolds, bone health transforms into a continuum of maintenance and adaptation. The bone remodeling process, orchestrated by osteoblasts and osteoclasts, ensures the continuous renewal of bone tissue. Factors such as nutrition, physical activity, and hormonal balance continue to exert their influence, impacting bone health throughout the lifespan.

In later years, particularly during postmenopausal stages, hormonal changes can accelerate bone loss, highlighting the importance of proactive measures such as weight-bearing exercises, a balanced diet, and medical interventions to preserve bone density. The journey of bone health encapsulates the resilience and adaptability of the skeletal system, emphasizing the significance of lifelong strategies to fortify and sustain this vital aspect of overall well-being.

CHAPTER TWO

What Causes Osteoporosis?

Osteoporosis, a condition characterized by weakened bones, is influenced by a combination of factors that disrupt the delicate balance between bone formation and resorption. Age is a primary contributor, as bone density tends to decrease naturally over time, especially in postmenopausal women due to declining estrogen levels. Genetic predispositions also play a role, with a family history of osteoporosis increasing the likelihood of its development.

Hormonal imbalances, particularly a reduction in estrogen during menopause, can accelerate bone loss. This hormone is crucial for maintaining bone density, and its decline can lead to increased osteoclast activity, resulting in greater bone resorption. In men, a decline in testosterone can have similar effects.

Lifestyle factors significantly contribute to osteoporosis risk. Inadequate nutrition, especially low calcium and vitamin D intake, compromises bone health. Sedentary lifestyles devoid of weight-bearing exercises contribute to reduced bone density. Smoking and excessive alcohol consumption are additional risk factors, as they can interfere with bone remodeling processes.

Certain medical conditions and medications can also induce osteoporosis. Conditions such as rheumatoid arthritis, hormonal disorders, and gastrointestinal disorders impact bone health. Long-term use of corticosteroids, anti-seizure medications, and some cancer treatments may also contribute to bone loss.

Understanding the multifaceted causes of osteoporosis is essential for proactive prevention and management strategies, emphasizing lifestyle modifications, adequate nutrition, and medical interventions to safeguard bone health.

Age and Gender Factors

Age and gender are pivotal factors influencing the development of osteoporosis, a condition characterized by diminished bone density and increased susceptibility to fractures. The aging process itself is a primary contributor, as bone mass tends to peak in the early 20s and gradually declines thereafter. The gradual reduction in bone density is more pronounced in women, especially after menopause when estrogen levels drop significantly. Estrogen plays a crucial role in maintaining bone density by inhibiting excessive bone resorption.

Postmenopausal women are at a heightened risk due to this hormonal shift. The first few years following menopause witness accelerated bone loss, particularly in trabecular bone, which is the spongy, inner part of the bone.

While age is a universal risk factor, gender differences are noteworthy. Women, generally having lower peak bone mass and a longer life expectancy, are more susceptible to osteoporosis. However, men are not exempt. Age-related bone loss in men becomes more apparent in later years, often accompanied by a decline in testosterone levels.

Understanding these age and gender factors is crucial for preventive measures and early detection. Regular bone density assessments, lifestyle modifications, and appropriate medical interventions become increasingly important as individuals age, offering a proactive approach to maintaining bone health and mitigating the impact of osteoporosis.

Genetic Predispositions

Genetic predispositions play a significant role in the development of osteoporosis, contributing to the variability in individual susceptibility to this bone-weakening condition. While bone health is influenced by a complex interplay of genetic and environmental factors, familial patterns often underscore a hereditary component in osteoporosis risk.

Certain genetic variations impact bone mineral density, bone structure, and the efficiency of bone remodeling processes. Variants in genes related to the synthesis and regulation of collagen, the main protein in bone, as well as those associated with vitamin D metabolism and estrogen receptors, can influence bone health.

Family history serves as a valuable indicator of genetic susceptibility. Individuals with parents or siblings who have experienced fractures or been diagnosed with osteoporosis may be at an increased risk due to shared genetic factors. Additionally, specific ethnic backgrounds may carry a higher prevalence of certain genetic variants associated with osteoporosis.

Understanding genetic predispositions allows for more targeted preventive measures and personalized interventions. While genes influence susceptibility, lifestyle factors such as nutrition, physical activity, and avoidance of detrimental habits remain crucial in mitigating the impact of genetic predispositions. Advances in genetic research continue to shed light on the intricate relationship between genetics and osteoporosis, paving the way for more precise risk assessments and tailored approaches to bone health management.

Hormonal Influences

Hormonal influences play a central role in the development and progression of osteoporosis, a condition characterized by bone loss and increased fracture risk. Estrogen, a key hormone in both men and women, plays a pivotal role in maintaining bone density. In postmenopausal women, the decline in estrogen levels accelerates bone resorption by osteoclasts, leading to a reduction in bone mass and increased susceptibility to fractures. The first few years after menopause are particularly critical for bone health due to the rapid decline in estrogen.

In men, testosterone is essential for bone health. Low testosterone levels, often associated with aging, can contribute to decreased bone density and an increased risk of osteoporosis. Additionally, conditions such as hypogonadism (low testosterone production) or certain hormonal treatments can influence bone health in men.

Thyroid hormones also impact bone metabolism. Both hyperthyroidism (excessive thyroid hormone production) and hypothyroidism (insufficient thyroid hormone production) can disrupt the delicate balance between bone formation and resorption, leading to bone loss.

Understanding hormonal influences on bone health is crucial for preventive measures and targeted interventions. Hormone replacement therapy (HRT) may be considered for postmenopausal women to mitigate the impact of estrogen decline. Maintaining hormonal balance through lifestyle choices and, when necessary, medical interventions is essential for preserving bone density and preventing osteoporosis.

Identifying Risk Factors

Identifying risk factors for osteoporosis is a crucial step in preventing and managing this bone-weakening condition. Several factors contribute to an individual's susceptibility, and recognizing them allows for targeted interventions and proactive measures.

1. Age and Gender: Aging is a primary risk factor, with bone density naturally decreasing over time. Postmenopausal women, due to a decline in estrogen, are particularly vulnerable.

2. Genetic Predisposition: Family history is indicative of genetic influences on bone health. Individuals with parents or siblings diagnosed with osteoporosis are at an increased risk.

3. Hormonal Changes: Hormones, such as estrogen and testosterone, play a vital role in maintaining bone density. Hormonal imbalances, especially during menopause or with low testosterone levels, can contribute to bone loss.

4. Nutritional Deficiencies: Inadequate intake of calcium and vitamin D compromises bone health. These nutrients are essential for bone mineralization and overall skeletal integrity.

5. Lifestyle Factors: Sedentary lifestyles, lack of weight-bearing exercises, smoking, and excessive alcohol consumption are significant contributors to osteoporosis risk.

6. Medical Conditions and Medications: Certain health conditions, like rheumatoid arthritis or gastrointestinal disorders, can impact bone health. Long-term use of medications like corticosteroids may also lead to bone loss.

Identifying these risk factors allows individuals and healthcare professionals to implement preventative strategies, including lifestyle modifications, nutritional interventions, and targeted medical treatments, reducing the likelihood of osteoporosis and its associated complications.

Lifestyle Contributors

Lifestyle choices exert a profound influence on bone health, and understanding the impact of lifestyle contributors is pivotal in the prevention and management of osteoporosis. Several aspects of daily living significantly affect bone density and overall skeletal strength.

1. Nutrition: Inadequate intake of essential nutrients, particularly calcium and vitamin D, undermines bone health. A diet rich in these nutrients, found in dairy products, leafy greens, and fortified foods, supports bone mineralization.

2. Physical Activity: Weight-bearing exercises, such as walking, jogging, and resistance training, stimulate bone formation and strengthen the skeletal system. Sedentary lifestyles, on the contrary, contribute to bone loss over time.

3. Smoking: Tobacco smoke contains toxins that interfere with the bone remodeling process, leading to decreased bone density. Smokers face an increased risk of fractures and impaired bone healing.

4. Alcohol Consumption: Excessive alcohol intake can hinder the body's ability to absorb calcium, disrupt hormone levels, and impair bone formation. Moderate alcohol consumption is advisable for maintaining bone health.

5. Body Weight: Maintaining a healthy body weight is essential for bone health. Both underweight and obesity can negatively impact bone density and increase the risk of fractures.

6. Avoidance of Falls: Taking precautions to prevent falls, especially in the elderly, is crucial. Falls can lead to fractures, and individuals with osteoporosis are more susceptible to bone injuries.

By addressing these lifestyle contributors, individuals can adopt habits that promote bone health, reduce the risk of osteoporosis, and contribute to overall well-being.

Medications and Other Influencing Elements

Medications and various influencing elements can significantly impact bone health, either by contributing to bone loss or by affecting the body's ability to maintain optimal bone density. Understanding these factors is crucial in assessing and managing the risk of osteoporosis.

1. Corticosteroids: Long-term use of corticosteroid medications, prescribed for conditions like rheumatoid arthritis and asthma, can lead to bone loss. These medications interfere with the bone remodeling process, resulting in decreased bone density and an elevated risk of fractures.

2. Hormone-Related Treatments: Certain hormonal treatments, including those for breast or prostate cancer, can induce hormonal imbalances that affect bone health. Similarly, treatments that induce menopause in women for medical reasons may contribute to bone loss.

3. Anticonvulsants: Some medications used to manage seizures (anticonvulsants) may interfere with the body's ability to absorb calcium, potentially leading to decreased bone density over time.

4. Gastrointestinal Disorders: Conditions affecting the gastrointestinal tract, such as celiac disease and inflammatory bowel disease, can impair nutrient absorption, including calcium. This, in turn, compromises bone health.

5. Weight Loss Medications: Certain medications used for weight loss may impact bone density. It's important to assess the potential effects on bone health when considering such treatments.

6. Medical Conditions: Chronic conditions like autoimmune disorders, hormonal imbalances, and chronic kidney disease can indirectly influence bone health by disrupting the delicate balance of bone formation and resorption.

Managing osteoporosis risk involves considering these influencing elements, and healthcare professionals work collaboratively with patients to evaluate the potential impact of medications and medical conditions on bone health. Adjustments to treatment plans and lifestyle interventions may be recommended to mitigate these effects and maintain optimal skeletal integrity.

CHAPTER THREE

The Role of Bone Density Testing

The role of bone density testing, also known as Dual-Energy X-ray Absorptiometry (DXA), is pivotal in the early detection, assessment, and monitoring of osteoporosis. This non-invasive imaging technique measures bone mineral density (BMD), providing valuable insights into the strength and density of bones, particularly in the hip and spine—common sites prone to osteoporotic fractures.

Bone density testing serves as a critical diagnostic tool, enabling healthcare professionals to identify individuals at risk of fractures due to compromised bone density. The results, often presented as T-scores, compare an individual's BMD to that of a healthy young adult, helping classify bone health status. A T-score of -1 or higher is considered normal, while scores between -1 and -2.5 indicate low bone density (osteopenia), and scores of -2.5 or lower are indicative of osteoporosis.

Beyond diagnosis, bone density testing plays a crucial role in assessing fracture risk and guiding treatment decisions. Regular monitoring with DXA scans allows healthcare providers to evaluate the effectiveness of interventions, such as lifestyle modifications or pharmacological treatments, and adjust management strategies accordingly.

In summary, bone density testing is a cornerstone in the comprehensive approach to osteoporosis management, facilitating early intervention, risk stratification, and personalized care plans aimed at preserving bone health and minimizing the impact of fractures.

Dual-Energy X-ray Absorptiometry (DXA)

Dual-Energy X-ray Absorptiometry (DXA) stands as a sophisticated and widely utilized imaging technique, revolutionizing the assessment of bone mineral density (BMD) and playing a pivotal role in the diagnosis and management of osteoporosis. This non-invasive and low-radiation technology employs two X-ray beams, each with different energy levels, to measure the attenuation of X-rays as they pass through bone and soft tissue.

DXA primarily focuses on key skeletal sites prone to osteoporotic fractures, predominantly the hip and spine. The results are expressed as T-scores, providing a quantitative measure of BMD by comparing an individual's bone density to that of a healthy young adult. T-scores serve as a critical diagnostic criterion, categorizing bone health into normal, osteopenia, or osteoporosis.

Beyond diagnosis, DXA scans play a crucial role in assessing fracture risk and guiding therapeutic decisions. The precision and reliability of DXA make it an invaluable tool for monitoring changes in bone density over time, evaluating treatment efficacy, and tailoring intervention strategies based on individual needs.

DXA's non-invasive nature, accuracy, and quick examination time have positioned it as the gold standard for bone density assessments, contributing significantly to the early detection and management of osteoporosis, ultimately enhancing patient outcomes and quality of life.

Interpreting Bone Density Results

Interpreting bone density results, typically provided as T-scores from Dual-Energy X-ray Absorptiometry (DXA) scans, is crucial for understanding an individual's bone health status and informing appropriate interventions. T-scores compare an individual's bone density to that of a healthy young adult, with a score of 0 indicating bone density comparable to the young adult reference.

1. Normal Bone Density (T-score > -1): A T-score of -1 or higher is considered normal, indicating bone density within the expected range for a young adult. No significant risk of fractures is associated with normal bone density.

2. Low Bone Density (T-score between -1 and -2.5): Scores between -1 and -2.5 suggest low bone density, a condition known as osteopenia. While not indicative of osteoporosis, it signifies reduced bone mass and an increased risk of fractures.

3. Osteoporosis (T-score ≤ -2.5): A T-score of -2.5 or lower indicates osteoporosis, characterized by significantly compromised bone density and an elevated risk of fractures. Immediate intervention and management strategies are often recommended.

Interpretation also considers additional factors such as age, gender, and medical history. Regular follow-up DXA scans enable healthcare professionals to monitor changes in bone density over time, assess treatment efficacy, and adjust interventions as needed, contributing to a comprehensive approach to bone health management.

Beyond Bone Density: Assessing Fracture Risk

Beyond assessing bone density, evaluating fracture risk involves a comprehensive analysis of multiple factors that contribute to skeletal strength and susceptibility to fractures. While Dual-Energy X-ray Absorptiometry (DXA) scans provide valuable information, other considerations play a crucial role in determining an individual's overall risk of fractures.

1. Clinical Risk Factors: Elements such as age, gender, family history of fractures, personal history of falls, and prior fracture occurrences contribute significantly to fracture risk. These clinical risk factors help refine the assessment beyond bone density alone.

2. Lifestyle Factors: Lifestyle choices, including physical activity, smoking, and alcohol consumption, influence bone health and fracture risk. Engaging in regular weight-bearing exercises, avoiding smoking, and moderating alcohol intake contribute to skeletal resilience.

3. Medical Conditions: Certain medical conditions, such as rheumatoid arthritis or hormonal disorders, can impact bone health and elevate fracture risk. Understanding and addressing these underlying conditions are essential for comprehensive fracture risk assessment.

4. Fall Risk: Assessing an individual's risk of falling is integral to determining fracture risk, especially in older adults. Factors like impaired balance, vision problems, and environmental hazards contribute to fall risk.

5. Medications: Certain medications, such as corticosteroids, anticonvulsants, and some treatments for chronic conditions, may contribute to bone loss and increase the likelihood of fractures.

Incorporating these factors into fracture risk assessments provides a more holistic understanding of an individual's vulnerability to fractures, guiding healthcare professionals in tailoring interventions and preventive strategies to enhance overall bone health and reduce the likelihood of fractures.

Integrating Clinical Assessment

Integrating clinical assessment into the evaluation of bone health involves a multidimensional approach, combining medical history, physical examinations, and diagnostic tools to derive a comprehensive understanding of an individual's skeletal status. Clinical assessment serves as a crucial complement to bone density testing, offering insights into factors that influence fracture risk and overall bone health.

1. Medical History: A thorough examination of an individual's medical history provides valuable information on factors such as previous fractures, family history of fractures, and the presence of medical conditions impacting bone health. Identifying these elements aids in tailoring interventions to specific needs.

2. Physical Examinations: Evaluating posture, balance, and musculoskeletal health through physical examinations contributes to assessing fall risk and identifying potential indicators of compromised bone integrity.

3. Laboratory Tests: Blood tests measuring markers of bone turnover, hormonal levels, and nutritional status offer additional insights into bone health. Elevated or decreased levels of specific markers may indicate underlying issues affecting bone metabolism.

4. Risk Factor Assessment: Integrating lifestyle factors, such as physical activity, smoking, and alcohol consumption, into the clinical assessment helps identify modifiable elements influencing bone health and fracture risk.

5. Medication Review: A review of medications, especially those known to impact bone density, guides healthcare professionals in understanding potential contributors to bone loss and tailoring management strategies accordingly.

By integrating clinical assessment components, healthcare providers can offer more personalized and targeted interventions, considering the holistic factors influencing bone health. This comprehensive approach enhances the precision of fracture risk assessment and supports the development of tailored strategies for optimizing skeletal strength and resilience.

Predictive Tools and Their Utility

Predictive tools in bone health serve as invaluable instruments for assessing and anticipating an individual's risk of developing osteoporosis and experiencing fractures. These tools amalgamate various clinical, lifestyle, and imaging data to generate risk estimates, aiding healthcare professionals in implementing preventive measures and personalized interventions.

1. Fracture Risk Assessment Tool (FRAX): FRAX is a widely utilized predictive tool that considers clinical risk factors, bone mineral density measurements, and country-specific fracture rates to estimate the 10-year probability of major osteoporotic fractures and hip fractures. It provides a quantitative and comprehensive assessment to guide treatment decisions.

2. Calcium and Vitamin D Intake Calculators: These tools help individuals and healthcare providers gauge daily calcium and vitamin D intake, essential for maintaining bone health. By assessing dietary habits and recommending necessary adjustments, these calculators contribute to preventive strategies.

3. Genetic Risk Assessment: Advances in genetic research have led to the development of tools that evaluate an individual's genetic predisposition to osteoporosis. By analyzing specific genetic markers, these tools offer insights into inherent risks, guiding early interventions and personalized care plans.

4. Fracture Risk Algorithms: These algorithms incorporate multiple risk factors, such as age, gender, bone density, and previous fractures, to predict the likelihood of future fractures. By identifying high-risk individuals, healthcare professionals can implement preventive measures and prioritize interventions.

The utility of predictive tools lies in their ability to inform evidence-based decision-making, tailor interventions to individual needs, and enhance the precision of fracture risk assessments, ultimately contributing to more effective strategies for osteoporosis prevention and management.

CHAPTER FOUR

Strategies for Prevention

Preventing osteoporosis involves a multifaceted approach, encompassing lifestyle modifications, nutritional interventions, and, when necessary, medical treatments. These strategies aim to optimize bone health, mitigate the risk of fractures, and foster overall well-being.

1. Nutrition: Adequate intake of calcium and vitamin D is fundamental for maintaining bone density. Calcium-rich foods like dairy products, leafy greens, and fortified foods, coupled with sufficient exposure to sunlight for vitamin D synthesis, support bone health.

2. Weight-Bearing Exercises: Engaging in regular weight-bearing exercises, such as walking, jogging, and resistance training, stimulates bone formation and enhances bone density. These activities contribute to overall musculoskeletal strength.

3. Avoidance of Smoking and Excessive Alcohol Consumption: Smoking has detrimental effects on bone remodeling, while excessive alcohol intake can hinder calcium absorption. Avoiding these habits is crucial for preserving bone health.

4. Fall Prevention: Implementing measures to prevent falls, especially in older adults, is vital for reducing the risk of fractures. This includes addressing environmental hazards, improving balance through exercises, and utilizing assistive devices when necessary.

5. Regular Health Check-ups: Periodic assessments of bone density, along with comprehensive health check-ups, help identify risk factors and guide preventive strategies. Early detection allows for timely interventions and the initiation of suitable treatments.

6. Medication When Necessary: For individuals at higher risk or with diagnosed osteoporosis, medications may be prescribed to enhance bone density and reduce fracture risk. These medications work in conjunction with lifestyle measures to optimize bone health.

By integrating these strategies into daily life, individuals can proactively preserve bone health, reduce the likelihood of osteoporosis, and maintain an active and independent lifestyle throughout their lifespan.

Building Bone Health Throughout Life

Building and maintaining bone health is a lifelong endeavor that requires a proactive and holistic approach. From childhood through the golden years, incorporating key strategies fosters skeletal resilience and reduces the risk of osteoporosis and fractures.

1. Early Childhood and Adolescence: Ensuring optimal bone development starts in early childhood. A balanced diet rich in calcium and vitamin D, along with regular physical activity, forms the foundation. The adolescent years, marked by rapid bone growth, benefit from weight-bearing exercises and healthy lifestyle habits.

2. Young Adulthood: Establishing and maintaining healthy habits, including a nutritious diet, regular exercise, and avoidance of harmful substances like tobacco and excessive alcohol, contribute to peak bone mass during young adulthood. These habits lay the groundwork for skeletal strength in later years.

3. Adulthood: Engaging in weight-bearing and muscle-strengthening exercises remains crucial in adulthood. Adequate intake of nutrients, including calcium and vitamin D, supports bone maintenance. Regular health check-ups, including bone density assessments, assist in monitoring bone health and identifying potential issues.

4. Menopause and Beyond: Women entering menopause face hormonal changes that affect bone density. Hormone replacement therapy, lifestyle modifications, and targeted interventions become vital in preserving bone health. For both genders, maintaining an active lifestyle, a nutrient-rich diet, and regular health assessments are essential in the later stages of life.

Building bone health throughout life involves a continuum of awareness, preventive measures, and adaptability to changing needs. By integrating these strategies across the lifespan, individuals can optimize bone health, promoting overall well-being and independence.

Childhood and Adolescent Years

The childhood and adolescent years represent a critical phase in building and nurturing bone health, laying the foundation for skeletal strength throughout life. During these formative years, the focus is on promoting optimal bone development and maximizing peak bone mass.

1. Nutrition: A balanced and nutrient-rich diet is fundamental. Adequate intake of calcium, found in dairy products, leafy greens, and fortified foods, is essential for bone mineralization. Vitamin D, obtained through sunlight exposure and dietary sources, supports calcium absorption.

2. Physical Activity: Weight-bearing exercises and activities that stimulate bone growth are crucial during childhood and adolescence. Sports, running, jumping, and resistance training contribute to bone density and strength. These activities foster not only skeletal health but also overall physical fitness.

3. Avoidance of Harmful Habits: Discouraging harmful habits, such as smoking and excessive alcohol consumption, is essential. These habits can interfere with the bone development process and compromise future bone health.

4. Regular Health Check-ups: Periodic health check-ups, including assessments of growth patterns and nutritional status, allow for early identification of potential issues. Addressing concerns promptly ensures appropriate interventions for optimal bone health.

Building bone health during childhood and adolescence is an investment in long-term well-being. These foundational years shape the trajectory of skeletal development, influencing the peak bone mass achieved in early adulthood and setting the stage for resilient bones throughout life.

Adult Life: Sustaining Healthy Habits

In adult life, sustaining healthy habits becomes paramount for maintaining and optimizing bone health. As the peak bone mass achieved in early adulthood begins to stabilize, it's crucial to focus on lifestyle choices that support skeletal resilience and prevent bone loss.

1. Nutrient-Rich Diet: Continuing a diet rich in calcium and vitamin D remains essential for maintaining bone density. Incorporating dairy products, leafy greens, and fortified foods ensures a sustained supply of these critical nutrients.

2. Regular Exercise: Weight-bearing and muscle-strengthening exercises are indispensable for skeletal maintenance. Activities like walking, jogging, resistance training, and flexibility exercises contribute to bone health, as well as overall physical fitness.

3. Avoidance of Harmful Substances: The avoidance of smoking and moderation in alcohol consumption remains crucial. These substances can negatively impact bone remodeling processes and compromise bone density.

4. Health Check-ups: Regular health check-ups, including bone density assessments, assist in monitoring bone health and identifying any changes or concerns. Early detection allows for timely interventions and adjustments to the management plan.

5. Fall Prevention: As individuals age, fall prevention becomes increasingly important. Measures such as ensuring a safe living environment, maintaining balance through exercises, and addressing vision or mobility issues contribute to fracture risk reduction.

By sustaining healthy habits into adulthood, individuals can fortify their bones, reduce the risk of osteoporosis, and support overall well-being. This proactive approach ensures that the foundation established in earlier years is reinforced, contributing to a robust and resilient skeletal system throughout life.

Lifestyle Modifications

Lifestyle modifications play a pivotal role in promoting and preserving bone health, offering practical and accessible strategies for individuals to adopt throughout their lives. These modifications encompass various aspects of daily living, influencing factors such as nutrition, physical activity, and habits that directly impact bone density and overall skeletal well-being.

1. Nutrition: Embracing a diet rich in calcium, vitamin D, and other essential nutrients is fundamental for bone health. Incorporating dairy products, leafy greens, nuts, and fortified foods ensures an adequate supply of key elements crucial for bone mineralization.

2. Physical Activity: Regular weight-bearing exercises, such as walking, jogging, and resistance training, stimulate bone formation and enhance overall musculoskeletal strength. Incorporating flexibility exercises also supports joint health.

3. Smoking Cessation: Quitting smoking is a crucial lifestyle modification as smoking has detrimental effects on bone remodeling, leading to decreased bone density and an increased risk of fractures.

4. Moderation in Alcohol Consumption: Limiting alcohol intake is advisable, as excessive alcohol consumption can interfere with calcium absorption and disrupt bone remodeling processes.

5. Fall Prevention: Taking measures to prevent falls, especially among older adults, includes addressing environmental hazards, maintaining balance through exercises, and utilizing assistive devices when necessary.

Lifestyle modifications are accessible, sustainable, and contribute significantly to maintaining optimal bone health. By incorporating these changes, individuals can proactively enhance skeletal resilience, reduce the risk of osteoporosis, and foster overall well-being throughout their lifespan.

Nutrition: Calcium and Vitamin D

Nutrition, particularly the intake of calcium and vitamin D, plays a central role in fostering robust bone health. These two essential nutrients are integral components in the bone mineralization process, influencing bone density and strength.

1. Calcium: As the primary mineral in bones, calcium is crucial for bone structure and integrity. Adequate calcium intake is necessary throughout life, but it is particularly vital during childhood and adolescence when bones are growing and developing. Dairy products, leafy green vegetables, nuts, and fortified foods are excellent sources of dietary calcium. Ensuring an adequate calcium supply supports optimal bone mineralization, reducing the risk of fractures and osteoporosis.

2. Vitamin D: Vitamin D facilitates the absorption of calcium from the intestines and promotes its incorporation into bones. While sunlight exposure triggers vitamin D synthesis in the skin, dietary sources such as fatty fish, fortified dairy products, and vitamin D supplements contribute to maintaining sufficient levels. In regions with limited sunlight, supplementation or dietary adjustments become crucial. Vitamin D deficiency can compromise calcium absorption, leading to weakened bones and an increased susceptibility to fractures.

Balancing calcium and vitamin D intake through a well-rounded diet or supplementation, when necessary, is a cornerstone of nutrition for bone health, promoting lifelong skeletal strength and resilience.

Weight-Bearing Exercises

Weight-bearing exercises are cornerstone components of a comprehensive approach to maintaining and enhancing bone health throughout life. These exercises involve supporting the body's weight against gravity, stimulating bone remodeling processes and contributing to skeletal strength and density.

1. Walking and Jogging: Simple yet effective, activities like walking and jogging provide low-impact weight-bearing benefits. These exercises encourage bone formation, especially in the weight-bearing bones of the lower extremities.

2. Resistance Training: Lifting weights or using resistance bands places stress on bones, prompting them to adapt by becoming denser and stronger. Strength training exercises targeting various muscle groups also contribute to bone health.

3. Dancing: Dance forms that involve weight-bearing, such as salsa or ballroom dancing, combine cardiovascular benefits with the advantages of weight-bearing exercises. The dynamic movements engage multiple muscle groups, fostering bone density.

4. Aerobic Exercise: Activities like aerobics, step aerobics, and jumping jacks are effective weight-bearing exercises. These high-impact activities create mechanical loading on bones, promoting bone mineralization and strength.

5. Hiking: Taking to the trails adds an element of incline and uneven terrain, intensifying the impact on weight-bearing bones. Hiking engages the lower body and spine, contributing to overall bone health.

Regular incorporation of weight-bearing exercises into a fitness routine is pivotal for optimizing bone health, reducing the risk of osteoporosis, and supporting overall musculoskeletal well-being. Always consult with healthcare professionals or fitness experts to ensure a safe and suitable exercise regimen based on individual needs and health conditions.

CHAPTER FIVE

The Role of Nutrition in Bone

Health

The role of nutrition in bone health is instrumental, with dietary choices significantly influencing bone density, strength, and overall skeletal integrity. Key nutrients play pivotal roles in bone formation, maintenance, and repair.

1. Calcium: As a fundamental component of bone mineralization, calcium is paramount for skeletal health. Dairy products like milk and yogurt, leafy green vegetables, nuts, and fortified foods are excellent sources. Insufficient calcium intake can compromise bone density, increasing the risk of fractures and osteoporosis.

2. Vitamin D: Essential for calcium absorption, vitamin D plays a synergistic role in bone health. Sunlight exposure triggers vitamin D synthesis in the skin, while dietary sources like fatty fish, fortified dairy products, and supplements contribute to maintaining adequate levels.

3. Vitamin K: Crucial for bone mineralization and the regulation of calcium within bones, vitamin K is found in green leafy vegetables, broccoli, and vegetable oils. Adequate vitamin K intake supports bone health.

4. Phosphorus: This mineral works in tandem with calcium to form the mineral matrix of bones. Meat, dairy, nuts, and whole grains are good sources of phosphorus, contributing to overall bone strength.

5. Magnesium: Involved in bone structure and mineralization, magnesium is present in nuts, seeds, whole grains, and green leafy vegetables. A balanced intake of magnesium supports bone health.

Balancing these nutrients through a diverse and nutrient-rich diet is essential for maintaining optimal bone health, preventing deficiencies, and reducing the risk of bone-related conditions throughout the lifespan.

Dietary Sources and Supplements

Dietary sources and supplements are crucial avenues for ensuring an adequate intake of essential nutrients that contribute to bone health. While a balanced diet should be the primary source of these nutrients, supplements can play a complementary role, especially when dietary intake is insufficient.

1. Dietary Sources:
  - Calcium: Dairy products such as milk and yogurt, leafy green vegetables, nuts, and fortified foods.
  - Vitamin D: Sunlight exposure triggers vitamin D synthesis. Dietary sources include fatty fish, fortified dairy products, and egg yolks.
  - Magnesium: Nuts, seeds, whole grains, leafy vegetables, and legumes.
  - Phosphorus:* Meat, dairy, nuts, whole grains, and fish.
  - Vitamin K: Green leafy vegetables, broccoli, and vegetable oils.

2. Supplements:
  - Calcium and Vitamin D: Commonly combined in supplements, especially for individuals with dietary deficiencies or limited sunlight exposure.

 - Magnesium, Phosphorus, and Vitamin K: Supplements are available, but these nutrients are often obtained adequately through a well-balanced diet.

Supplements should be used judiciously and under the guidance of healthcare professionals. While they can fill nutritional gaps, relying on whole foods for nutrient intake offers additional benefits beyond bone health, contributing to overall well-being. Dietary diversity remains a cornerstone for achieving optimal bone strength and maintaining a comprehensive spectrum of essential nutrients.

Crafting a Bone-Friendly Diet

Crafting a bone-friendly diet involves intentional choices to ensure a consistent and balanced intake of nutrients crucial for bone health. A diet rich in the following elements contributes to optimal bone density, strength, and overall skeletal resilience.

1. Calcium-Rich Foods: Incorporate dairy products such as milk, yogurt, and cheese. Non-dairy sources like leafy greens (kale, broccoli), tofu, and fortified plant-based milk are excellent alternatives.

2. Vitamin D Sources: Prioritize foods rich in vitamin D, including fatty fish (salmon, mackerel), egg yolks, and fortified dairy or plant-based milk. Sunlight exposure is also crucial for vitamin D synthesis.

3. Magnesium-Containing Foods: Include nuts (almonds, cashews), seeds (sunflower, pumpkin), whole grains, and green leafy vegetables to meet magnesium needs.

4. Phosphorus-Packed Foods: Consume a variety of protein-rich foods like meat, dairy, nuts, and legumes to ensure sufficient phosphorus intake.

5. Leafy Greens for Vitamin K: Incorporate green leafy vegetables like kale, spinach, and broccoli, which are rich in vitamin K.

6. Balanced Protein Intake: Include sources of lean protein, such as poultry, fish, beans, and legumes, to support overall bone health.

7. Limit Caffeine and Soda: Excessive caffeine and soda consumption can interfere with calcium absorption. Moderation is key.

8. Stay Hydrated: Water is essential for overall health, including the health of bones. Ensure adequate hydration to support optimal bodily functions.

Crafting a bone-friendly diet involves diversity, balance, and attention to individual nutritional needs. Consulting with a healthcare professional or a registered dietitian can help tailor dietary choices to specific requirements for optimal bone health.

Meal Plans and Recipes

Designing meal plans and recipes that prioritize bone health involves incorporating a variety of nutrient-rich foods to ensure a well-rounded intake of essential elements like calcium, vitamin D, magnesium, and more. Here's a blueprint for crafting bone-friendly meals:

1. Breakfast:
   - Calcium and Vitamin D: Start with a bowl of fortified cereal with milk or yogurt. Add a side of sliced oranges for vitamin C, aiding calcium absorption.

2. Lunch:
   - Leafy Greens and Protein: Create a salad with spinach, kale, and broccoli. Add grilled salmon or tofu for protein. Dress with olive oil for vitamin K.

3. Snack:

- Nuts and Seeds: Snack on a handful of almonds and pumpkin seeds. These provide magnesium and phosphorus essential for bone health.

4. Dinner:
- Lean Protein and Whole Grains: Opt for grilled chicken or beans as a protein source. Serve with quinoa or brown rice, offering phosphorus and magnesium.

5. Vegetables:
- Colorful Variety: Include a mix of colorful vegetables in each meal. Bell peppers, carrots, and sweet potatoes contribute vitamins and minerals.

6. Dessert:
- Fruit Parfait: Layer yogurt with fresh berries and granola. This provides calcium, vitamin D, and antioxidants.

Recipes can be adapted to suit individual preferences and dietary restrictions. It's crucial to focus on a diverse and nutrient-dense approach, ensuring each meal contributes to overall bone health. Consulting with a nutrition professional can help tailor meal plans to specific needs and preferences.

Meal Plans and Recipes

Creating well-rounded meal plans with bone health in mind involves thoughtful selection of nutrient-rich foods that support optimal bone density and overall well-being. Below is a detailed guide along with sample recipes for a day.

Day's Meal Plan for Bone Health:

Breakfast:
- Meal: Greek Yogurt Parfait
  - Ingredients: Greek yogurt, mixed berries, granola, and a drizzle of honey.
  - Nutritional Highlights: Greek yogurt provides calcium and protein; berries offer antioxidants, and granola adds whole grains.

Lunch:
- Meal: Salmon and Quinoa Salad
  - Ingredients: Grilled salmon, quinoa, mixed greens, cherry tomatoes, cucumbers, and a lemon vinaigrette.
  - Nutritional Highlights: Salmon provides vitamin D and omega-3 fatty acids; quinoa offers protein, magnesium, and phosphorus.

Snack:
- Meal: Trail Mix
  - Ingredients: Almonds, walnuts, pumpkin seeds, and dried apricots.

- Nutritional Highlights: Nuts and seeds contribute magnesium, phosphorus, and healthy fats.

Dinner:
- Meal: Chickpea and Spinach Stew
  - Ingredients: Chickpeas, spinach, tomatoes, garlic, onions, and vegetable broth.
  - Nutritional Highlights: Chickpeas provide protein and phosphorus; spinach adds calcium and vitamin K.

Vegetables:
- Side Dish: Roasted Vegetables
  - Ingredients: Colorful bell peppers, zucchini, and carrots.
  - Nutritional Highlights: These vegetables provide vitamins and minerals, including vitamin C for collagen production.

Dessert:
- Treat: Chia Seed Pudding
  - Ingredients: Chia seeds, almond milk, vanilla extract, and fresh berries.
  - Nutritional Highlights: Chia seeds are rich in calcium and omega-3 fatty acids.

Key Considerations:
- Calcium Intake: Ensure a variety of dairy or fortified plant-based milk products.

- Vitamin D: Include fatty fish, egg yolks, or fortified foods.
- Magnesium and Phosphorus: Nuts, seeds, legumes, and whole grains are excellent sources.

Key Note: Adapt portion sizes based on individual needs and consult with a healthcare professional or nutritionist for personalized guidance.

Creating bone-friendly meal plans involves a balance of nutrients and a diverse range of foods. These recipes emphasize key elements supporting bone health, promoting a holistic approach to overall well-being.

Balancing Nutritional Intake

Balancing nutritional intake is essential for overall health, and it plays a critical role in promoting bone health. Achieving equilibrium among various nutrients ensures that the body receives the necessary elements for optimal bone density, strength, and resilience.

1. Calcium and Vitamin D: Striking a balance between these two is crucial. While dairy products, leafy greens, and fortified foods contribute calcium, vitamin D from sunlight exposure and dietary sources like fatty fish supports calcium absorption.

2. Magnesium and Phosphorus: Nuts, seeds, whole grains, and legumes are excellent sources of magnesium and phosphorus. Balancing their intake helps maintain bone mineralization and structural integrity.

3. Protein: Adequate protein intake is vital for bone health. Incorporating lean meats, fish, legumes, and dairy products provides essential amino acids necessary for bone formation.

4. Vitamins K and C: Leafy greens, broccoli, and colorful vegetables supply vitamin K, while fruits such as oranges and strawberries contribute vitamin C. These vitamins play roles in bone mineralization and collagen synthesis.

5. Fats: Including healthy fats from sources like avocados, nuts, and olive oil supports overall bone health and nutrient absorption.

Achieving a well-rounded and balanced diet involves diversity and moderation. Consulting with a registered dietitian or healthcare professional can provide personalized guidance, ensuring that nutritional intake aligns with individual needs and supports long-term bone health.

CHAPTER SIX

Beyond Prevention: Managing

Osteoporosis

Beyond prevention, effectively managing osteoporosis involves a comprehensive approach that addresses both lifestyle modifications and medical interventions. As a chronic condition characterized by reduced bone density and increased fracture risk, managing osteoporosis aims to slow its progression, alleviate symptoms, and enhance overall quality of life.

1. Medication: Various medications are available to treat osteoporosis. Bisphosphonates, denosumab, and hormone therapy are common options that work by either slowing bone loss or promoting bone formation. These medications are prescribed based on individual health profiles and specific needs.

2. Calcium and Vitamin D Supplementation: Adequate calcium and vitamin D intake remain crucial in managing osteoporosis. Supplements may be recommended, especially when dietary sources are insufficient, to support bone health.

3. Weight-Bearing Exercises: While high-impact exercises may be limited in individuals with osteoporosis, low-impact weight-bearing exercises, along with strength training, can help maintain bone density and improve overall muscle strength and balance.

4. Fall Prevention: Implementing measures to prevent falls becomes paramount. This includes home safety assessments, vision checks, and exercises to improve balance and coordination, reducing the risk of fractures.

5. Regular Monitoring: Regular bone density testing allows healthcare professionals to monitor changes in bone density over time and adjust treatment plans as needed.

Collaboration with healthcare providers is crucial in tailoring a management plan that addresses the unique aspects of each individual's osteoporosis. This comprehensive approach ensures a holistic strategy that combines medical interventions with lifestyle modifications for effective long-term management.

Medications for Osteoporosis

Medications for osteoporosis are diverse and tailored to address specific aspects of bone health, aiming to slow bone loss, promote bone formation, and reduce the risk of fractures. Here are some common medications used in the management of osteoporosis:

1. Bisphosphonates: This class of drugs, including alendronate and risedronate, inhibits bone resorption by osteoclasts, preserving bone density. They are often prescribed as oral tablets or intravenous infusions.

2. Denosumab: A monoclonal antibody, denosumab, targets a protein involved in bone breakdown. Administered as a subcutaneous injection, it reduces bone resorption, enhancing bone density.

3. Hormone Therapy: Estrogen or a combination of estrogen and progestin may be prescribed for postmenopausal women to mitigate bone loss. Hormone therapy is administered with caution due to associated risks and benefits.

4. Selective Estrogen Receptor Modulators (SERMs):
Medications like raloxifene mimic the effects of estrogen
on bone tissue, offering protection against bone loss in
postmenopausal women.

5. Teriparatide and Abaloparatide: These drugs are
forms of parathyroid hormone that stimulate bone
formation. They are administered as daily injections and
are reserved for specific cases due to their cost and
mode of administration.

6. Calcitonin: Derived from salmon, calcitonin helps
regulate calcium and phosphate levels, with potential
bone-preserving effects. It is available as a nasal spray or
injection.

Individual treatment plans are determined based on
factors such as age, gender, fracture risk, and overall
health. Healthcare professionals tailor medication
regimens to provide optimal bone health benefits while
considering potential side effects and individual needs.
Regular monitoring and adjustments are essential to
ensure effective management of osteoporosis.

Bisphosphonates and Other Pharmacological Options

Bisphosphonates are a class of medications widely used in the management of osteoporosis, offering effective strategies to slow bone loss and reduce the risk of fractures. These drugs, such as alendronate, risedronate, and zoledronic acid, work by inhibiting bone resorption, suppressing the activity of osteoclasts, the cells responsible for breaking down bone tissue.

Alendronate and risedronate are typically administered orally as tablets, while zoledronic acid is delivered intravenously. Regular use of bisphosphonates has demonstrated improvements in bone density and a reduction in fractures, particularly in postmenopausal women.

Beyond bisphosphonates, several other pharmacological options play crucial roles in osteoporosis management:

1. Denosumab: A monoclonal antibody that inhibits bone resorption by targeting a protein involved in bone breakdown. Administered as a subcutaneous injection, denosumab provides an alternative for those unable to tolerate bisphosphonates.

2. Teriparatide and Abaloparatide: These medications, analogs of parathyroid hormone, stimulate bone formation and are administered through daily injections. They are considered in specific cases, such as severe osteoporosis or intolerance to other treatments.

3. Hormone Therapy: Estrogen or a combination of estrogen and progestin may be prescribed, particularly for postmenopausal women, to mitigate bone loss. However, the use of hormone therapy is carefully considered due to associated risks and benefits.

Individualized treatment plans, considering factors like age, gender, and overall health, are essential in determining the most suitable pharmacological options for managing osteoporosis. Regular monitoring and collaboration with healthcare professionals ensure optimal treatment efficacy and safety.

Benefits, Risks, and Side Effects

The use of medications in osteoporosis management, such as bisphosphonates and other pharmacological options, entails both benefits and potential risks, along with the possibility of side effects.

Benefits:
1. Increased Bone Density: Bisphosphonates and other medications contribute to increased bone density, reducing the risk of fractures in individuals with osteoporosis.
2. Fracture Risk Reduction: Pharmacological interventions can significantly decrease the likelihood of fractures, particularly in high-risk populations, enhancing overall skeletal health.
3. Pain Relief: Medications may alleviate bone pain associated with fractures or bone deterioration, improving the quality of life for individuals with osteoporosis.

Risks:
1. Atypical Fractures: Prolonged use of bisphosphonates has been associated with rare atypical fractures, especially in the femur. This risk must be weighed against the benefits, particularly in long-term usage.
2. Gastrointestinal Issues: Some individuals may experience gastrointestinal discomfort or irritation when taking bisphosphonates orally.
3. Renal Impairment: Long-term use of certain medications, particularly intravenous bisphosphonates, may pose a risk of renal impairment.

Side Effects:

1. Flu-like Symptoms: Some individuals may experience flu-like symptoms after bisphosphonate infusion.
2. Skin Reactions: Skin reactions at the injection site are possible with medications administered subcutaneously.
3. Hormone Therapy Risks: Estrogen-based therapies, while beneficial for bone health, carry potential risks, including an increased risk of breast cancer and cardiovascular issues.

The decision to use these medications involves careful consideration of an individual's overall health, lifestyle, and risk factors. Healthcare professionals play a crucial role in assessing the benefits and risks, tailoring treatment plans, and monitoring for potential side effects to ensure the safest and most effective osteoporosis management.

The Role of Hormone Replacement Therapy (HRT)

Hormone Replacement Therapy (HRT) has been a longstanding option for managing osteoporosis, particularly in postmenopausal women. The role of HRT lies in supplementing declining hormone levels, primarily estrogen, which plays a crucial role in maintaining bone density. Here are key aspects of the role of HRT in osteoporosis management:

1. Estrogen and Bone Health:
  - Estrogen plays a pivotal role in regulating bone turnover by inhibiting bone resorption. During menopause, estrogen levels decline, leading to accelerated bone loss and an increased risk of fractures.

2. Prevention of Bone Loss:
  - HRT aims to mitigate bone loss by providing supplemental estrogen, thereby preserving bone density. This can reduce the risk of osteoporotic fractures, particularly in the spine and hips.

3. Individualized Approach:
  - The decision to use HRT is highly individualized and depends on factors such as a woman's age, overall health, and the presence of other risk factors. It is often considered for postmenopausal women who are at an increased risk of fractures.

4. Risks and Benefits:
  - The use of HRT is associated with both benefits, such as improved bone health, and risks, including an increased risk of breast cancer and cardiovascular issues. The decision to undergo HRT involves careful consideration of these factors, and it is usually reserved for women with significant bone health concerns.

5. Regular Monitoring:
   - Women on HRT are regularly monitored by healthcare professionals to assess its effectiveness, adjust dosage if necessary, and evaluate potential side effects or risks.

While HRT remains a viable option for some women, it is crucial to weigh its benefits against potential risks, and the decision to use HRT should be made collaboratively between a woman and her healthcare provider based on individual health needs and circumstances.

Considerations and Alternatives

When contemplating the use of hormone replacement therapy (HRT) or other medications for osteoporosis, several considerations and alternative approaches should be carefully weighed to ensure the most suitable and effective management strategy.

Considerations:

1. Individual Health Profile: The decision to use HRT or other medications should be based on an individual's overall health, medical history, and specific risk factors.

Conditions such as breast cancer, cardiovascular issues, or a history of blood clots may influence the choice of treatment.

2. Duration of Use: The optimal duration of HRT is a critical consideration. Short-term use to manage acute symptoms may differ from long-term use for osteoporosis prevention. Regular reassessment with healthcare professionals is essential.

3. Monitoring and Side Effects: Regular monitoring of bone density and potential side effects is crucial. It allows healthcare providers to adjust treatment plans, assess the medication's effectiveness, and address any emerging concerns.

Alternatives:

1. Lifestyle Modifications: Emphasizing lifestyle changes, including a nutrient-rich diet, weight-bearing exercises, and fall prevention strategies, can significantly contribute to bone health.

2. Other Medications: Depending on individual circumstances, bisphosphonates, denosumab, or selective estrogen receptor modulators (SERMs) may be considered as alternatives to HRT.

3. Natural Approaches: Some individuals explore natural alternatives such as herbal supplements or dietary changes. However, the efficacy and safety of these approaches require further research and consultation with healthcare professionals.

Balancing considerations and exploring alternatives involves open communication between individuals and their healthcare providers. By carefully evaluating health profiles and preferences, a tailored osteoporosis management plan can be crafted, optimizing both effectiveness and safety.

Collaborative Approaches with Healthcare Providers

Collaborative approaches with healthcare providers are integral to effective osteoporosis management, ensuring a personalized and well-informed strategy that aligns with individual health needs. Here are key aspects of a collaborative approach:

1. Comprehensive Assessment:
   - Healthcare providers conduct thorough assessments, considering factors such as bone density, medical history, lifestyle, and potential risk factors. This comprehensive

evaluation forms the basis for tailored management plans.

2. Informed Decision-Making:
   - Collaborative decision-making empowers individuals to actively participate in choosing the most suitable treatment options. Healthcare providers provide detailed information about benefits, risks, and alternatives, fostering informed choices.

3. Regular Monitoring:
   - Ongoing collaboration involves regular monitoring of bone health through tests like dual-energy X-ray absorptiometry (DXA) scans. Periodic assessments enable adjustments to treatment plans based on individual responses and changes in health status.

4. Lifestyle Recommendations:
   - Healthcare providers offer guidance on lifestyle modifications, emphasizing the importance of a nutrient-rich diet, weight-bearing exercises, fall prevention strategies, and overall healthy habits.

5. Addressing Concerns:
   - Open communication allows individuals to express concerns, preferences, or any adverse effects experienced during treatment. Healthcare providers can then promptly address these concerns, ensuring the continuity of care.

6. Shared Goals:

   - Establishing shared goals between individuals and healthcare providers creates a collaborative framework. These goals may include improving bone density, reducing fracture risk, and enhancing overall quality of life.

Collaborative approaches foster a sense of partnership, enhancing the effectiveness of osteoporosis management. By actively involving individuals in their care and leveraging the expertise of healthcare providers, these collaborative efforts contribute to the development of tailored, patient-centered strategies that optimize bone health outcomes.

CHAPTER SEVEN

Dietary Factors in Osteoporosis

Management

Dietary factors play a pivotal role in the management of osteoporosis, influencing bone health through the supply of essential nutrients that contribute to bone density and overall skeletal integrity.

1. Calcium-Rich Foods:
   - Adequate calcium intake is crucial for bone mineralization. Dairy products like milk, yogurt, and cheese are primary sources, but non-dairy alternatives such as fortified plant-based milk, leafy greens, and nuts are also valuable contributors.

2. Vitamin D Sources:

- Vitamin D is essential for calcium absorption and bone health. Fatty fish like salmon, mackerel, fortified dairy products, and exposure to sunlight are key sources to ensure sufficient vitamin D levels.

3. Magnesium and Phosphorus:
- Nuts, seeds, whole grains, and leafy vegetables provide magnesium and phosphorus, supporting bone structure and mineralization.

4. Vitamin K-Rich Foods:
- Leafy greens such as kale and spinach are rich in vitamin K, which plays a role in bone mineralization and helps regulate calcium within bones.

5. Balanced Protein Intake:
- Including lean protein sources like poultry, fish, beans, and legumes supports overall bone health by providing essential amino acids necessary for bone formation.

6. Limiting Caffeine and Soda:
- Excessive caffeine and soda consumption can interfere with calcium absorption. Moderation in these beverages contributes to better bone health.

A well-balanced and nutrient-rich diet, coupled with other lifestyle modifications, forms a holistic approach to osteoporosis management. Consulting with healthcare professionals or registered dietitians can help tailor dietary plans to individual needs, optimizing the impact of nutrition on bone health.

Tailoring Nutrition for Ongoing Management

Tailoring nutrition for ongoing osteoporosis management involves adapting dietary choices to meet individual needs, ensuring a consistent supply of essential nutrients crucial for bone health. Here are key considerations for personalized nutrition in the ongoing management of osteoporosis:

1. Individual Nutrient Needs:
   - Assessing individual nutrient requirements, including calcium, vitamin D, magnesium, phosphorus, and vitamin K, is essential. Tailoring intake based on age, gender, health status, and dietary preferences ensures optimal bone health support.

2. Customizing Calcium Intake:
   - Individualizing calcium intake involves choosing a variety of calcium-rich foods, considering factors like lactose intolerance or dietary restrictions. Incorporating dairy or fortified plant-based alternatives, along with leafy greens and nuts, contributes to balanced calcium intake.

3. Personalized Vitamin D Strategies:
   - Addressing vitamin D needs involves balancing sunlight exposure, dietary sources, and potential supplementation. Individuals with limited sun exposure or specific risk factors may benefit from personalized vitamin D plans.

4. Dietary Modifications:
   - Adapting the diet to address specific health conditions or concerns is crucial. For example, individuals with renal issues may need adjustments to phosphorus intake.

5. Regular Monitoring:
   - Periodic assessments of bone health and nutritional status allow for adjustments in dietary plans. Monitoring ensures that nutritional strategies align with changing health needs over time.

Collaboration with healthcare professionals or registered dietitians is pivotal in tailoring ongoing nutrition plans. Customizing dietary approaches based on individual circumstances ensures that nutrition remains a key component of effective, personalized osteoporosis management.

Adjusting Diets Alongside Medication

Adjusting diets alongside osteoporosis medications is a crucial aspect of comprehensive management, ensuring optimal support for bone health while considering the specific requirements and potential interactions associated with pharmaceutical interventions.

1. Calcium and Vitamin D Synergy:
 - Medications like bisphosphonates often work synergistically with calcium and vitamin D. Adjusting diets to include adequate calcium-rich foods and optimizing vitamin D levels can enhance the effectiveness of these medications.

2. Dietary Calcium Considerations:
 - Some osteoporosis medications may require specific conditions for optimal absorption. For instance, bisphosphonates are best absorbed on an empty stomach, and calcium-rich foods or supplements should be consumed at least two hours apart from these medications to avoid interference.

3. Addressing Potential Side Effects:
 - Dietary adjustments can help mitigate potential side effects of medications. For example, individuals experiencing gastrointestinal discomfort with oral

bisphosphonates may benefit from dietary modifications that reduce acidity.

4. Nutrient-Rich Diets:

   - Ensuring a nutrient-rich diet supports overall bone health and addresses potential nutritional deficiencies associated with certain medications. This includes a diverse range of fruits, vegetables, whole grains, and protein sources.

5. Monitoring Nutrient Intake:

   - Regular monitoring of nutrient intake, especially calcium and vitamin D levels, allows for adjustments to dietary plans based on individual responses to medications and changing health needs over time.

A collaborative approach involving healthcare professionals, including dietitians and prescribing physicians, is essential to fine-tune dietary plans alongside osteoporosis medications. This ensures that nutrition complements the therapeutic goals of the medications and contributes to comprehensive osteoporosis management.

Monitoring Nutrient Levels

Monitoring nutrient levels is a crucial aspect of osteoporosis management, ensuring that individuals receive adequate amounts of essential nutrients to support bone health while avoiding potential imbalances or deficiencies. Here are key considerations for monitoring nutrient levels in the context of osteoporosis:

1. Calcium Intake:
   - Regular assessment of dietary calcium intake is vital. Monitoring calcium-rich food consumption and considering supplements when necessary help maintain optimal bone mineralization.

2. Vitamin D Status:
   - Periodic checks of vitamin D levels are essential, especially in individuals with limited sun exposure or specific risk factors. Adjusting dietary sources and potential supplementation ensures adequate vitamin D support for calcium absorption.

3. Magnesium and Phosphorus Levels:
   - Monitoring magnesium and phosphorus levels helps maintain a balanced mineral environment for bone health. Nutrient-rich foods like nuts, seeds, and whole grains contribute to these minerals.

4. Vitamin K Assessment:
   - Regular evaluation of vitamin K levels is important, as this nutrient plays a role in bone mineralization. Leafy

greens and other vitamin K-rich foods contribute to overall bone health.

5. Protein Intake:

- Assessing protein intake, particularly sources rich in essential amino acids, helps support bone formation. Regular monitoring ensures that protein needs align with individual health and medication considerations.

6. Regular Bone Density Testing:

- Dual-energy X-ray absorptiometry (DXA) scans provide valuable information about bone density changes. Monitoring these results alongside nutrient levels allows for a holistic understanding of bone health and the effectiveness of nutritional interventions.

Collaboration between healthcare professionals and registered dietitians facilitates ongoing nutrient monitoring, enabling personalized adjustments to dietary plans and optimizing nutritional support for individuals managing osteoporosis.

CHAPTER EIGHT

Maintaining Quality of Life

Maintaining a high quality of life while managing osteoporosis involves a holistic approach that encompasses physical, emotional, and social well-being. Here are key considerations to ensure a fulfilling and vibrant life despite the challenges of osteoporosis:

1. Physical Activity:
  - Engaging in regular, bone-friendly exercises such as walking, swimming, or gentle weight-bearing activities helps maintain muscle strength, flexibility, and balance. Customized exercise routines contribute to overall physical well-being.

2. Nutrient-Rich Diet:
  - Adhering to a balanced and nutrient-rich diet, with a focus on calcium, vitamin D, and other essential nutrients, supports bone health and overall vitality.

Dietary choices should be enjoyable and align with individual preferences.

3. Fall Prevention:

- Implementing strategies to prevent falls, such as creating a safe living environment, using assistive devices if necessary, and practicing balance exercises, reduces the risk of fractures and enhances confidence in daily activities.

4. Emotional Well-being:

- Cultivating emotional resilience through activities like mindfulness, meditation, or participating in support groups fosters mental well-being. Emotional health contributes to a positive outlook on life despite the challenges posed by osteoporosis.

5. Social Engagement:

- Maintaining social connections with friends, family, or community groups provides emotional support and combats feelings of isolation. Staying socially active contributes to a sense of belonging and joy.

6. Regular Health Check-ups:

- Regular check-ups with healthcare professionals, including bone density testing and assessments of nutrient levels, ensure that osteoporosis management aligns with individual health needs. This proactive approach supports overall well-being.

Adopting a multifaceted approach that combines physical activity, a balanced diet, emotional resilience, and social engagement contributes to a high quality of life for individuals managing osteoporosis. It empowers individuals to lead fulfilling lives while proactively addressing their bone health and overall wellness.

Coping with Emotional Aspects

Coping with the emotional aspects of osteoporosis is integral to holistic well-being, considering the potential impact of this condition on mental health and overall quality of life. Managing the emotional challenges associated with osteoporosis involves adopting coping strategies that foster resilience and a positive mindset:

1. Education and Understanding:
   - Gaining knowledge about osteoporosis and its management helps individuals understand their condition, fostering a sense of control and empowerment. This knowledge equips individuals to make informed decisions about their health.

2. Emotional Support:

- Seeking emotional support from friends, family, or support groups provides a crucial outlet for expressing feelings, fears, and frustrations. Knowing that one is not alone in facing these challenges can alleviate emotional burdens.

3. Mental Health Practices:

- Incorporating mental health practices such as mindfulness, meditation, or deep-breathing exercises helps manage stress and anxiety associated with osteoporosis. These practices promote emotional well-being and resilience.

4. Goal Setting:

- Setting realistic and achievable goals, both short-term and long-term, provides a sense of purpose and accomplishment. Celebrating small victories contributes to a positive outlook.

5. Professional Counseling:

- Seeking professional counseling or therapy can be beneficial for those facing emotional distress related to their condition. Professional guidance provides tools to cope with anxiety, depression, or feelings of uncertainty.

6. Advocacy and Empowerment:

- Becoming an advocate for one's own health and engaging in decision-making processes with healthcare professionals empowers individuals to take an active role in their osteoporosis management. This sense of control positively impacts emotional well-being.

Addressing the emotional aspects of osteoporosis requires a comprehensive approach that combines self-education, social support, mental health practices, and professional guidance. By acknowledging and actively coping with emotional challenges, individuals can navigate the emotional terrain of osteoporosis with resilience and a positive mindset.

Support Networks and Resources

Building a robust support network and accessing valuable resources are essential components of effectively managing osteoporosis. These networks offer emotional encouragement, information, and practical assistance, enhancing overall well-being:

1. Support Groups:
  - Joining osteoporosis support groups provides a platform for individuals to share experiences, exchange information, and receive emotional support from others facing similar challenges. This fosters a sense of community and reduces feelings of isolation.

2. Healthcare Professionals:

- Establishing strong connections with healthcare professionals, including primary care physicians, endocrinologists, and orthopedic specialists, ensures ongoing guidance and monitoring. These professionals offer valuable insights into treatment options, lifestyle adjustments, and overall osteoporosis management.

3. Family and Friends:

- Informing and involving family and friends in the journey of osteoporosis management creates a strong support foundation. Loved ones can provide emotional support, assist with daily activities, and contribute to a positive environment.

4. Educational Resources:

- Accessing reputable educational resources, both online and offline, offers valuable information on osteoporosis management, treatment options, and lifestyle modifications. Reliable sources empower individuals to make informed decisions about their health.

5. National Osteoporosis Foundations:

- National and local osteoporosis foundations often provide educational materials, support services, and community events. These organizations serve as valuable resources for staying informed and connected within the osteoporosis community.

6. Online Platforms:

- Utilizing online platforms, forums, and social media groups dedicated to osteoporosis enables individuals to connect with a broader community, share experiences, and access a wealth of information and support.

Establishing and maintaining a strong support network, coupled with accessing diverse resources, contributes to a more positive and informed osteoporosis management experience. These networks offer not only practical assistance but also emotional encouragement, fostering resilience and overall well-being.

Strategies for Independence and Mobility

Maintaining independence and mobility is paramount for individuals managing osteoporosis. Strategic approaches empower individuals to navigate daily life confidently while mitigating the risk of fractures and enhancing overall well-being:

1. Regular Exercise:

- Incorporating weight-bearing exercises, balance training, and flexibility exercises into a regular routine strengthens muscles and bones, improving overall mobility and reducing the risk of falls.

2. Assistive Devices:

   - Using assistive devices such as canes, walkers, or handrails provides additional support, particularly in environments where stability may be a concern. These aids enhance mobility and reduce the risk of accidents.

3. Home Safety Modifications:

   - Adapting the home environment by removing potential hazards, installing grab bars in bathrooms, and ensuring proper lighting improves safety and allows for greater independence at home.

4. Fall Prevention Strategies:

   - Implementing fall prevention strategies, including regular eye check-ups, wearing appropriate footwear, and minimizing clutter, significantly reduces the risk of falls that can lead to fractures.

5. Medication Management:

   - Adhering to medication regimens as prescribed by healthcare professionals is crucial. Proper medication management contributes to bone health and minimizes the risk of complications.

6. Balanced Nutrition:

- Following a nutrient-rich diet, including adequate calcium and vitamin D, supports bone health and overall well-being. Proper nutrition contributes to strength and resilience, enhancing independence.

7. Regular Health Check-ups:
- Scheduling regular health check-ups, including bone density testing, ensures that osteoporosis is effectively managed. Monitoring overall health allows for timely adjustments to lifestyle and treatment plans.

By integrating these strategies into daily life, individuals with osteoporosis can maintain independence and mobility, fostering a sense of control over their health and well-being. These approaches, when personalized to individual needs, contribute to a fulfilling and active lifestyle despite the challenges posed by osteoporosis.

Adaptive Techniques

Adaptive techniques are invaluable tools for individuals managing osteoporosis, offering practical solutions to overcome challenges and enhance daily living. These techniques empower individuals to adapt to their specific needs, fostering independence and improving overall quality of life:

1. Body Mechanics and Posture:
 - Learning proper body mechanics and maintaining good posture is crucial to prevent unnecessary strain on bones and muscles. This includes techniques for lifting, sitting, and standing to reduce the risk of fractures.

2. Joint Protection Techniques:
 - Implementing joint protection techniques helps minimize stress on joints, particularly in areas vulnerable to fractures. This may involve using ergonomic tools or modifying activities to reduce joint impact.

3. Mobility Aids:
 - Utilizing mobility aids such as canes, walkers, or crutches provides additional support, enhancing stability and reducing the risk of falls. These aids facilitate safer and more confident movement.

4. Ergonomic Home Modifications:
 - Making ergonomic adjustments at home, such as installing grab bars, using elevated seats, or arranging furniture for easy navigation, promotes a safer environment and facilitates independent living.

5. Energy Conservation Techniques:
 - Practicing energy conservation techniques involves pacing activities, prioritizing tasks, and taking breaks to

avoid fatigue. This helps individuals manage daily responsibilities without overexertion.

6. Adaptive Clothing and Footwear:
   - Choosing adaptive clothing with easy fastenings and comfortable footwear with proper support minimizes physical strain and makes dressing and walking more manageable.

7. Assistive Devices:
   - Integrating assistive devices like reachers, long-handled tools, or jar openers simplifies daily tasks and reduces the need for strenuous movements, contributing to joint and bone health.

By incorporating adaptive techniques into daily routines, individuals with osteoporosis can navigate challenges more effectively, fostering independence and maintaining a fulfilling and active lifestyle. These techniques, often tailored to individual needs, empower individuals to overcome limitations and live with confidence.

Physical Activity and Safe Practices

Engaging in physical activity is a cornerstone of osteoporosis management, promoting bone strength, muscle health, and overall well-being. However, safe practices are paramount to prevent injuries and fractures. Here's a guide on incorporating physical activity while prioritizing safety:

1. Consult with Healthcare Professionals:
   - Before starting any exercise regimen, consult with healthcare professionals, especially if there are existing health concerns or osteoporosis-related complications. They can provide personalized recommendations based on individual health conditions.

2. Focus on Weight-Bearing Exercises:
   - Weight-bearing exercises, such as walking, dancing, and stair climbing, promote bone density and muscle strength. Incorporate these activities into a regular routine, gradually increasing intensity to avoid strain.

3. Include Strength Training:
   - Strength training, with a focus on resistance exercises, enhances muscle mass and supports bone health. Utilize resistance bands or light weights, gradually increasing as strength improves.

4. Emphasize Balance and Flexibility:

   - Incorporate exercises that enhance balance and flexibility, reducing the risk of falls. Activities like yoga or tai chi contribute to stability and overall mobility.

5. Modify High-Risk Activities:
   - Modify or avoid activities that pose a higher risk of falls or fractures. High-impact activities like jumping or intense aerobics may need to be adjusted to lower-impact alternatives.

6. Practice Safe Body Mechanics:
   - Implement safe body mechanics during activities and daily tasks. Avoid excessive bending, twisting, or heavy lifting to prevent unnecessary stress on bones and joints.

7. Gradual Progression:
   - Gradually progress in intensity and duration of exercises to allow the body to adapt. Sudden or excessive increases in activity may lead to injuries.

By combining physical activity with safe practices, individuals with osteoporosis can maintain and improve their overall health while minimizing the risk of fractures. Regular assessments and adaptations to the exercise routine ensure that activities align with individual capabilities and contribute to long-term bone health.

CHAPTER NINE

Integrating Long-Term Habits

Integrating long-term habits is essential for individuals managing osteoporosis, providing a sustainable framework for maintaining bone health and overall well-being. Establishing these habits involves adopting a holistic approach that encompasses lifestyle, nutrition, and consistent self-care practices:

1. Regular Physical Activity:
  - Make regular, weight-bearing exercises a habit. Incorporate activities like walking, swimming, or gentle aerobics into daily routines to promote bone density, muscle strength, and flexibility.

2. Balanced Nutrition:
  - Cultivate a habit of consuming a nutrient-rich diet that includes adequate calcium, vitamin D, and other essential nutrients for bone health. Regularly reassess

and adjust dietary habits to meet changing nutritional needs.

3. Medication Adherence:
 - If prescribed medications, develop a routine for adherence. Taking medications as prescribed by healthcare professionals ensures consistent support for bone health.

4. Fall Prevention Measures:
 - Integrate fall prevention strategies into daily life. Ensure a safe home environment, use assistive devices if needed, and practice activities that enhance balance to reduce the risk of falls.

5. Regular Health Check-ups:
 - Make routine health check-ups a habit. Regular assessments, including bone density testing and nutrient level monitoring, allow for proactive adjustments to long-term management plans.

6. Stress Management:
 - Incorporate stress management techniques, such as mindfulness, meditation, or hobbies, as regular habits. Reducing stress contributes to overall well-being and indirectly supports bone health.

7. Social Engagement:

- Foster a habit of social engagement. Maintaining connections with friends, family, or support groups provides emotional support and a sense of community.

By integrating these habits into daily life, individuals with osteoporosis can create a sustainable and supportive framework for long-term management. Consistency and commitment to these practices contribute to not only managing osteoporosis effectively but also cultivating a holistic and fulfilling lifestyle.

Sustainable Nutrition

Sustainable nutrition is a cornerstone of long-term osteoporosis management, emphasizing a balanced and environmentally conscious approach to food choices. This involves adopting dietary practices that promote both personal health and the health of the planet:

1. Plant-Based Emphasis:
   - Prioritize plant-based foods, including fruits, vegetables, legumes, and whole grains. These foods are rich in essential nutrients while generally requiring fewer environmental resources than animal-based products.

2. Locally Sourced and Seasonal Foods:

- Choose locally sourced and seasonal foods whenever possible. This not only supports local economies but also reduces the carbon footprint associated with the transportation of goods.

3. Sustainable Protein Sources:

- Opt for sustainable protein sources such as legumes, nuts, seeds, and responsibly sourced fish. These choices contribute to a nutrient-rich diet while minimizing the environmental impact.

4. Mindful Consumption:

- Practice mindful consumption by avoiding food waste. Plan meals, store food properly, and use leftovers creatively to minimize environmental impact and maximize nutritional intake.

5. Limit Processed Foods:

- Minimize the consumption of highly processed foods and sugary beverages. Choosing whole, unprocessed foods not only supports bone health but also aligns with sustainable dietary principles.

6. Water Conservation:

- Conserve water by making mindful choices, such as reducing meat consumption (which has a higher water footprint) and choosing water-efficient cooking methods.

7. Education and Advocacy:
   - Stay informed about sustainable food practices and advocate for policies that support a more sustainable food system. This includes supporting local farmers, reducing food waste, and promoting environmentally friendly agriculture.

Sustainable nutrition for osteoporosis management extends beyond personal health to encompass broader environmental considerations. By making conscious and informed choices, individuals can contribute to both their well-being and the sustainability of the planet.

Exercise Routines Across the Lifespan

Adopting and adapting exercise routines across the lifespan is crucial for promoting bone health and overall well-being, especially in the context of osteoporosis management. Here's a guide on age-appropriate exercise strategies:

Childhood and Adolescence:
   - Emphasize weight-bearing activities like running, jumping, and sports to promote optimal bone development during these critical growth years.

Encourage a variety of physical activities to foster lifelong habits.

Adult Life:
   - Incorporate a mix of aerobic exercises, strength training, and flexibility exercises. Weight-bearing activities continue to be essential, and resistance training helps maintain muscle mass and bone density. Activities such as walking, cycling, and moderate-intensity workouts are beneficial.

Older Adults:
   - Focus on exercises that improve balance, coordination, and flexibility to prevent falls. Weight-bearing exercises remain important, but modifications may be needed based on individual health conditions. Low-impact activities like swimming and tai chi can be beneficial.

Seniors:
   - Adapt exercise routines to accommodate changing abilities and potential health concerns. Gentle, weight-bearing activities, resistance training, and flexibility exercises remain important. Incorporate activities that improve mobility and reduce the risk of fractures.

Consistency and adaptability are key across all life stages. Tailoring exercise routines to individual capabilities and health conditions ensures a lifelong commitment to bone health and overall fitness. Always consult with healthcare professionals before starting or modifying exercise regimens, especially in the presence of osteoporosis or related concerns.

Creating a Bone-Friendly Living Environment

Creating a bone-friendly living environment is essential for individuals managing osteoporosis, fostering safety, and minimizing the risk of fractures. Consider these key elements for a supportive living space:

1. Adequate Lighting:
   - Ensure well-lit spaces to enhance visibility and reduce the risk of trips and falls, especially in hallways, staircases, and commonly used areas.

2. Non-Slip Flooring:
   - Use non-slip rugs and mats in areas prone to moisture, such as bathrooms and kitchens. Secure carpets and ensure that flooring is even and free from obstacles.

3. Furniture Arrangement:

- Arrange furniture to allow for clear pathways and easy navigation. Avoid clutter to minimize the risk of tripping.

4. Grab Bars and Handrails:
- Install grab bars in bathrooms and handrails along staircases to provide additional support and stability.

5. Adequate Seating:
- Ensure that chairs and sofas provide proper support and are at a height that allows for easy sitting and standing, reducing the risk of falls.

6. Assistive Devices:
- Consider using assistive devices such as canes or walkers if needed. Make sure these devices are easily accessible and in good working condition.

7. Organization and Accessibility:
- Keep frequently used items within reach to avoid excessive reaching or bending. Consider organizing spaces to minimize the need for strenuous movements.

8. Temperature Control:
- Maintain a comfortable temperature to prevent stiffness and discomfort. Adequate heating in colder seasons is crucial for joint and muscle health.

9. Regular Maintenance:

- Regularly inspect and maintain the home environment. Fix loose handrails, repair uneven flooring, and address any potential hazards promptly.

10. Emergency Preparedness:
- Have an emergency plan in place, including easy access to a phone and contact information for emergency services. Consider using medical alert systems for added safety.

Creating a bone-friendly living environment involves thoughtful planning and adjustments to daily surroundings. By incorporating these measures, individuals with osteoporosis can minimize the risk of accidents, promote safety, and enhance their overall quality of life within their homes.

Home Modifications for Safety

Home modifications for safety are paramount for individuals managing osteoporosis, helping to minimize the risk of falls and fractures. Consider these essential modifications to create a safer living environment:

1. Bathroom Safety:

- Install grab bars near toilets and in showers or tubs to provide stability. Consider non-slip mats to prevent accidents on wet surfaces.

2. Adequate Lighting:

- Ensure sufficient lighting in all areas, especially staircases, hallways, and entrances. Well-lit spaces contribute to improved visibility and reduce the risk of tripping.

3. Non-Slip Flooring:

- Choose flooring options that are non-slip, particularly in bathrooms and kitchens. Secure area rugs with non-slip backing or remove them altogether.

4. Handrails:

- Install handrails along staircases and ramps. This provides essential support and promotes safer movement between different levels of the home.

5. Height-Accessible Items:

- Arrange frequently used items within easy reach to minimize reaching or bending. This includes kitchen utensils, clothing, and toiletries.

6. Doorway Accessibility:

- Ensure that doorways are wide enough to accommodate mobility aids if necessary. Consider lever-style door handles for easier use.

7. Adequate Seating:
   - Provide sturdy and comfortable seating throughout the home. Chairs and sofas should be at a height that allows for easy sitting and standing.

8. Clear Pathways:
   - Arrange furniture and other items to create clear pathways. Remove clutter to reduce the risk of tripping.

9. Emergency Preparedness:
   - Have an emergency plan in place, including accessible exits and easy access to a phone or emergency alert system.

By implementing these home modifications, individuals can significantly enhance the safety and accessibility of their living spaces, creating an environment that supports their osteoporosis management journey.

Awareness of Surroundings

Maintaining awareness of surroundings is a fundamental aspect of managing osteoporosis and preventing accidents. Developing a heightened sense of environmental awareness helps individuals navigate their daily lives with greater safety and confidence:

1. Mindful Movement:
- Practice mindful movement by paying attention to steps, uneven surfaces, or potential hazards. This includes being cautious on stairs, avoiding rushed movements, and adapting to changes in terrain.

2. Environmental Scanning:
- Regularly scan the environment for potential risks, such as loose rugs, wet surfaces, or obstacles in pathways. Proactive observation allows for timely adjustments to ensure safety.

3. Adequate Lighting:
- Ensure that spaces are well-lit, as proper lighting enhances visibility and reduces the likelihood of trips and falls. Adequate illumination is especially crucial in high-traffic areas.

4. Footwear Awareness:
- Choose appropriate footwear that provides support and stability. Avoid slippery or unsupportive shoes, especially on uneven or unfamiliar surfaces.

5. Seating Arrangement:

- Be mindful of the arrangement of chairs and furniture to create clear pathways. This reduces the risk of accidental collisions or tripping hazards.

6. Weather Considerations:
   - Consider weather conditions and adjust movement accordingly. Be cautious on slippery surfaces, such as icy sidewalks or wet floors, and adapt footwear and pace accordingly.

7. Home Modifications:
   - Implement home modifications for safety, including handrails, non-slip surfaces, and accessible pathways. A consciously designed living environment contributes to overall safety awareness.

By cultivating awareness of surroundings, individuals with osteoporosis can proactively manage their risk of accidents, promote a safer living environment, and maintain a higher quality of life. Regular mindfulness in daily activities contributes to a sense of control and confidence in navigating various settings.

CHAPTER TEN

Current Osteoporosis Research

Landscape

As of my last knowledge update in January 2022, the osteoporosis research landscape has been dynamic, with ongoing efforts to advance understanding, prevention, and treatment of this bone-related condition. It's essential to note that developments may have occurred since then, and I recommend checking the latest literature for the most recent information.

Researchers continue to explore various aspects of osteoporosis, including:

1. Novel Therapies:

- Investigating new pharmacological treatments and therapeutic approaches to enhance bone health and reduce fracture risk.

2. Precision Medicine:

- Exploring personalized or precision medicine strategies to tailor osteoporosis interventions based on an individual's genetic, lifestyle, and health factors.

3. Biomarkers:

- Identifying reliable biomarkers for early detection, prognosis, and monitoring of osteoporosis progression.

4. Lifestyle Interventions:

- Studying the impact of lifestyle modifications, such as diet, exercise, and other behavioral changes, on bone health and fracture prevention.

5. Bone Microarchitecture:

- Delving into the microarchitecture of bones to better understand the structural changes associated with osteoporosis.

6. Fracture Risk Assessment:

- Improving tools and methods for assessing fracture risk, including the integration of advanced imaging techniques and predictive modeling.

The ongoing research aims to provide a deeper understanding of osteoporosis, leading to more effective prevention and treatment strategies. Staying informed about the latest research findings is crucial for advancing clinical care and improving outcomes for individuals affected by osteoporosis.

Emerging Treatments and Therapies

In the ever-evolving landscape of osteoporosis research and treatment, several emerging therapies and approaches show promise in addressing the complexities of this bone-related condition. As of my last knowledge update in January 2022, here are some trends in emerging treatments:

1. Anabolic Agents:
   - Anabolic therapies, which stimulate bone formation, are gaining attention. These agents aim to increase bone density and strength by promoting the activity of bone-forming cells.

2. Combination Therapies:
   - Researchers are exploring the effectiveness of combining different medications to target multiple aspects of bone health. This approach may involve

combining antiresorptive agents with anabolic agents for a synergistic effect.

3. Biologic Therapies:
   - Biologic drugs that target specific pathways involved in bone metabolism are under investigation. These therapies aim to modulate the immune system and influence bone turnover.

4. Gene Therapy:
   - Gene-based interventions are being explored to enhance bone formation or inhibit excessive bone resorption. These approaches seek to address the genetic factors contributing to osteoporosis.

5. Mesenchymal Stem Cell Therapy:
   - Mesenchymal stem cell-based therapies are being researched for their potential to regenerate bone tissue and improve bone quality.

While these emerging treatments hold promise, it's essential to note that research is ongoing, and these therapies may still be in various stages of development or clinical trials. Continued advancements in understanding osteoporosis at the molecular and genetic levels are likely to shape the future of targeted and personalized treatment approaches. Individuals are encouraged to stay informed about the latest developments through reputable medical sources.

Promising Developments

Promising developments in the field of osteoporosis research and treatment are offering new avenues for more effective management of this bone-related condition. Here are some noteworthy advances:

1. Targeted Therapies:
- The identification of specific molecular targets involved in bone metabolism has paved the way for targeted therapies. Drugs that selectively modulate these targets aim to address bone loss more precisely.

2. Digital Health and Monitoring:
- The integration of digital health technologies, such as wearable devices and smartphone applications, allows for real-time monitoring of physical activity, nutrition, and medication adherence, contributing to more comprehensive osteoporosis management.

3. Patient-Centered Approaches:
- Increasing emphasis on patient-centered care involves tailoring treatment plans to individual needs, preferences, and lifestyle factors. This approach aims to

enhance patient engagement and improve long-term adherence to treatment regimens.

4. Collaborative Care Models:
   - Collaborative care models involve interdisciplinary approaches, bringing together healthcare professionals, including rheumatologists, endocrinologists, and primary care physicians, to optimize osteoporosis management and fracture prevention.

These promising developments underscore the ongoing commitment to advancing osteoporosis research and patient care. As research continues to unfold, these innovations hold the potential to significantly improve outcomes for individuals affected by osteoporosis.

CHAPTER ELEVEN

Taking Charge of Your Bone Health

Taking charge of your bone health is a proactive and empowering approach to preventing and managing osteoporosis. Here are key steps to foster strong and resilient bones throughout life:

1. Education and Awareness:
   - Stay informed about osteoporosis, its risk factors, and preventive measures. Knowledge empowers you to make informed decisions about your lifestyle and healthcare.

2. Balanced Nutrition:
   - Adopt a nutrient-rich diet rich in calcium, vitamin D, and other essential nutrients. Incorporate dairy products, leafy greens, and fortified foods to support bone health.

3. Regular Physical Activity:

- Engage in weight-bearing exercises, strength training, and activities that enhance balance and flexibility. Regular physical activity is fundamental for maintaining bone density and overall well-being.

4. Lifestyle Modifications:
- Implement lifestyle changes such as quitting smoking and limiting alcohol intake. These adjustments positively impact bone health and reduce the risk of fractures.

5. Bone Density Testing:
- Discuss with healthcare professionals the necessity and frequency of bone density testing based on individual risk factors. Early detection allows for timely interventions.

6. Medication Adherence:
- If prescribed medications, adhere to the recommended regimen. Consistent use of medications supports bone health and reduces the risk of fractures.

7. Fall Prevention:
- Implement measures to prevent falls, such as home modifications, regular vision check-ups, and awareness of surroundings. Minimizing falls is crucial for avoiding fractures.

By taking an active role in your bone health, you contribute to a resilient skeletal system, reducing the impact of osteoporosis and promoting overall well-being. Regular communication with healthcare professionals ensures personalized guidance for effective prevention and management strategies.

Personalized Action Plan

Crafting a personalized action plan for bone health empowers individuals to address specific risk factors and tailor interventions for optimal results. Here's a guide to developing a personalized strategy:

1. Risk Assessment:
   - Begin with a comprehensive risk assessment, considering factors such as age, gender, family history, lifestyle, and existing health conditions. This forms the foundation for a targeted action plan.

2. Nutrient-Rich Diet:
   - Tailor your diet to include foods rich in calcium, vitamin D, and other essential nutrients. A nutritionist can help create a personalized meal plan aligning with your specific dietary needs and preferences.

3. Physical Activity Goals:

- Set achievable physical activity goals based on your current fitness level and health status. Consult with a fitness professional to develop a well-rounded exercise routine, encompassing weight-bearing exercises, strength training, and balance-enhancing activities.

4. Medication Management:

- If prescribed medications, work closely with healthcare professionals to ensure adherence and address any concerns or side effects. Personalizing medication management is crucial for optimizing bone health.

5. Lifestyle Modifications:

- Identify and implement lifestyle modifications suited to your circumstances. This may include smoking cessation, limiting alcohol intake, and creating a home environment that minimizes the risk of falls.

6. Regular Monitoring:

- Establish a schedule for regular monitoring, including bone density testing and overall health check-ups. Periodic assessments allow for adjustments to the action plan based on your evolving health status.

A personalized action plan considers your unique health profile, aligning interventions with individual needs and preferences. Regular communication with healthcare professionals ensures ongoing support and guidance for effective bone health management.

Advocating for Bone Health in Your Community

Advocating for bone health in your community is a proactive way to raise awareness, promote preventive measures, and create a supportive environment for individuals at risk of osteoporosis. Here are effective ways to be a bone health advocate:

1. Education Initiatives:
   - Organize workshops, webinars, or community events to educate people about osteoporosis, its risk factors, and preventive strategies. Share information on nutrition, exercise, and lifestyle choices that support bone health.

2. Collaboration with Local Organizations:
   - Partner with local healthcare organizations, community centers, and schools to integrate bone health awareness into existing programs. Collaborative efforts amplify the reach and impact of advocacy initiatives.

3. Engage in Social Media Campaigns:

- Utilize social media platforms to share informative content, infographics, and success stories related to bone health. Encourage community members to share their experiences and engage in conversations.

4. Support Groups:
  - Establish or participate in local support groups for individuals dealing with osteoporosis. These groups provide a platform for sharing insights, experiences, and emotional support.

5. Workplace Wellness Programs:
  - Advocate for bone health within workplaces by promoting wellness programs that include ergonomic considerations, educational seminars, and fitness initiatives.

6. Policy Advocacy:
  - Engage with local policymakers to advocate for policies that support bone health, such as creating safe public spaces, promoting healthy lifestyle initiatives, and integrating bone health education into school curricula.

By actively advocating for bone health, you contribute to the well-being of your community, fostering a culture of prevention and support. Your efforts can positively impact individuals at risk of osteoporosis and inspire community-wide initiatives for better bone health.

CONCLUSION

In conclusion, understanding and actively managing osteoporosis is crucial for maintaining a high quality of life, especially as we age. This comprehensive guide has explored the intricacies of osteoporosis, covering its definition, impact on daily life, and the dynamic nature of bone health. Delving into the causes, risk factors, and identification of osteoporosis has provided a foundation for both prevention and effective management.

Recognizing the importance of bone density testing and the role of various influencing elements, from lifestyle contributors to medications, forms a vital part of this journey. Beyond bone density, exploring predictive tools, preventive strategies, and personalized action plans empowers individuals to take charge of their bone health.

From childhood and adolescence through adulthood and into senior years, this guide has underscored the significance of tailored exercise routines, nutrition, and lifestyle modifications. The evolving research landscape, promising developments, and emerging treatments offer hope for improved outcomes in the future.

As advocates for bone health, individuals can make a lasting impact on their communities, fostering awareness, education, and supportive environments. Ultimately, the journey to optimal bone health is a lifelong commitment, and by integrating knowledge, proactive measures, and community engagement, we can collectively build a foundation for stronger, more resilient bones and healthier lives.

Encouraging a Proactive Approach to Bone Health

Encouraging a proactive approach to bone health is paramount for individuals of all ages, as it fosters resilience and reduces the risk of osteoporosis-related complications. Firstly, cultivating awareness about the dynamic nature of bones and their susceptibility to various factors like aging, genetics, and lifestyle choices is essential. Education empowers individuals to make informed decisions and embrace preventive measures.

Promoting regular physical activity, including weight-bearing exercises and strength training, contributes significantly to bone density and overall well-being. The emphasis on balanced nutrition, with a focus on calcium and vitamin D-rich foods, supports bone health from an early age.

Regular check-ups and bone density testing are integral components of a proactive approach, allowing for early detection and timely interventions. Lifestyle modifications, such as quitting smoking and moderating alcohol intake, contribute to overall health and play a crucial role in preventing bone loss.

By fostering a proactive mindset, individuals become advocates for their own well-being, taking charge of their bone health journey. This not only benefits individuals but also contributes to the creation of communities that prioritize preventive measures, education, and support, ultimately building a foundation for healthier, more resilient lives.